The Medical Health Checklist1

Copyright: Published in the United States by Rita L. Spears
Published March 2017

ISBN-13: 978-1544253725

ISBN-10: 1544253729

NAME: _____

Personal Information

Full Name: _____ **SSN:** __-__-__

Address: _____ **DOB:** __/__/__

City/ST/Zip: _____ **Phone:** (___) ___-___

In Case of Emergency

Contact: _____ **Donor:** Y/N

Home #: (___) ___-___ **Directives:** _____

Mobile #: (___) ___-___ _____

Insurance Carrier

Company: _____ **ID #:** _____

Employer: _____ **Group #:** _____

Habits

Smoker: _____ **Drinks/WK:** _____

Blood Type: _____ **Allergies:** _____

Current Medications

Pharmacy Contact Number: (___) ___-___

Name	Description	Dosage	Purpose

Vitamins/Food Supplements

Name	Description	Dosage	Purpose

Known Conditions, Events, and Previous Surgeries

Date	Event

NAME: _____

Personal Information

Full Name:	_____	SSN:	__-__-__
Address:	_____	DOB:	__/__/__
City/ST/Zip:	_____	Phone:	(___) ___-___

In Case of Emergency

Contact:	_____	Donor:	Y/N
Home #:	(___) ___-___	Directives:	_____
Mobile #:	(___) ___-___		_____

Insurance Carrier

Company:	_____	ID #:	_____
Employer:	_____	Group #:	_____

Habits

Smoker:	_____	Drinks/WK:	_____
Blood Type:	_____	Allergies:	_____

Current Medications

Pharmacy Contact Number: (___) ___-___

Name	Description	Dosage	Purpose

Vitamins/Food Supplements

Name	Description	Dosage	Purpose

Known Conditions, Events, and Previous Surgeries

Date	Event

NAME: _____

Personal Information

Full Name:	_____	SSN:	__-__-__
Address:	_____	DOB:	__/__/__
City/ST/Zip:	_____	Phone:	(__) ___-__

In Case of Emergency

Contact:	_____	Donor:	Y/N
Home #:	(__) ___-__	Directives:	_____
Mobile #:	(__) ___-__		_____

Insurance Carrier

Company:	_____	ID #:	_____
Employer:	_____	Group #:	_____

Habits

Smoker:	_____	Drinks/WK:	_____
Blood Type:	_____	Allergies:	_____

Current Medications

Pharmacy Contact Number: (___) ___-__

Name	Description	Dosage	Purpose

Vitamins/Food Supplements

Name	Description	Dosage	Purpose

Known Conditions, Events, and Previous Surgeries

Date	Event

NAME: _____

Personal Information

Full Name: _____   SSN: __ - __ - __
Address: _____   DOB: __/__/__
City/ST/Zip: _____   Phone: (__) __-__

In Case of Emergency

Contact: _____   Donor: Y/N
Home #: (__) __-__   Directives: _____
Mobile #: (__) __-__   _____

Insurance Carrier

Company: _____   ID #: _____
Employer: _____   Group #: _____

Habits

Smoker: _____   Drinks/WK: _____
Blood Type: _____   Allergies: _____

Current Medications

Pharmacy Contact Number: (__) __-__

Name	Description	Dosage	Purpose

Vitamins/Food Supplements

Name	Description	Dosage	Purpose

Known Conditions, Events, and Previous Surgeries

Date	Event

NAME: _____

Personal Information

Full Name: _____   SSN: __-__-__

Address: _____   DOB: __/__/__

City/ST/Zip: _____   Phone: (___) ___-___

In Case of Emergency

Contact: _____   Donor: Y/N

Home #: (___) ___-___   Directives: _____

Mobile #: (___) ___-___   _____

Insurance Carrier

Company: _____   ID #: _____

Employer: _____   Group #: _____

Habits

Smoker: _____   Drinks/WK: _____

Blood Type: _____   Allergies: _____

Current Medications

Pharmacy Contact Number: (___) ___-___

Name	Description	Dosage	Purpose

Vitamins/Food Supplements

Name	Description	Dosage	Purpose

Known Conditions, Events, and Previous Surgeries

Date	Event

NAME: _____

Personal Information

Full Name:	_____	SSN:	__-__-__
Address:	_____	DOB:	__/__/__
City/ST/Zip:	_____	Phone:	(___) ___-___

In Case of Emergency

Contact:	_____	Donor:	Y/N
Home #:	(___) ___-___	Directives:	_____
Mobile #:	(___) ___-___		_____

Insurance Carrier

Company:	_____	ID #:	_____
Employer:	_____	Group #:	_____

Habits

Smoker:	_____	Drinks/WK:	_____
Blood Type:	_____	Allergies:	_____

Current Medications

Pharmacy Contact Number: (___) ___-___

Name	Description	Dosage	Purpose

Vitamins/Food Supplements

Name	Description	Dosage	Purpose

Known Conditions, Events, and Previous Surgeries

Date	Event

NAME: _____

Personal Information

Full Name: _____   SSN: __-__-__

Address: _____   DOB: __/__/__

City/ST/Zip: _____   Phone: (___) ___-__

In Case of Emergency

Contact: _____   Donor: Y/N

Home #:   (___) ___-__   Directives: _____

Mobile #:   (___) ___-__   _____

Insurance Carrier

Company: _____   ID #:   _____

Employer: _____   Group #:   _____

Habits

Smoker: _____   Drinks/WK: _____

Blood Type: _____   Allergies: _____

Current Medications

Pharmacy Contact Number: (___) ___-__

Name	Description	Dosage	Purpose

Vitamins/Food Supplements

Name	Description	Dosage	Purpose

Known Conditions, Events, and Previous Surgeries

Date	Event

NAME: _____

Personal Information

Full Name: _____	**SSN:** __-__-__
Address: _____	**DOB:** __/__/__
City/ST/Zip: _____	**Phone:** (___) ___-___

In Case of Emergency

Contact: _____	**Donor:** Y/N
Home #: (___) ___-___	**Directives:** _____
Mobile #: (___) ___-___	_____

Insurance Carrier

Company: _____	**ID #:** _____
Employer: _____	**Group #:** _____

Habits

Smoker: _____	**Drinks/WK:** _____
Blood Type: _____	**Allergies:** _____

Current Medications

Pharmacy Contact Number: (___) ___-___

Name	Description	Dosage	Purpose

Vitamins/Food Supplements

Name	Description	Dosage	Purpose

Known Conditions, Events, and Previous Surgeries

Date	Event

NAME: _____

Personal Information

Full Name: _____ SSN: __ __ - __ __ - __ __

Address: _____ DOB: __ / __ / __

City/ST/Zip: _____ Phone: (___) ___-___

In Case of Emergency

Contact: _____ Donor: Y/N

Home #: (___) ___-___ Directives: _____

Mobile #: (___) ___-___ _____

Insurance Carrier

Company: _____ ID #: _____

Employer: _____ Group #: _____

Habits

Smoker: _____ Drinks/WK: _____

Blood Type: _____ Allergies: _____

Current Medications

Pharmacy Contact Number: (___) ___-___

Name	Description	Dosage	Purpose

Vitamins/Food Supplements

Name	Description	Dosage	Purpose

Known Conditions, Events, and Previous Surgeries

Date	Event

NAME: _____

Personal Information

Full Name:	_____	SSN:	__-__-__
Address:	_____	DOB:	__/__/__
City/ST/Zip:	_____	Phone:	(__) __-__

In Case of Emergency

Contact:	_____	Donor:	Y/N
Home #:	(__) __-__	Directives:	_____
Mobile #:	(__) __-__		_____

Insurance Carrier

Company:	_____	ID #:	_____
Employer:	_____	Group #:	_____

Habits

Smoker:	_____	Drinks/WK:	_____
Blood Type:	_____	Allergies:	_____

Current Medications

Pharmacy Contact Number: (__) __-__

Name	Description	Dosage	Purpose

Vitamins/Food Supplements

Name	Description	Dosage	Purpose

Known Conditions, Events, and Previous Surgeries

Date	Event

NAME: _____

Personal Information

Full Name:	_____	**SSN:**	__-__-__
Address:	_____	**DOB:**	__/__/__
City/ST/Zip:	_____	**Phone:**	(___) ___-__

In Case of Emergency

Contact:	_____	**Donor:**	Y/N
Home #:	(___) ___-__	**Directives:**	_____
Mobile #:	(___) ___-__		_____

Insurance Carrier

Company:	_____	**ID #:**	_____
Employer:	_____	**Group #:**	_____

Habits

Smoker:	_____	**Drinks/WK:**	_____
Blood Type:	_____	**Allergies:**	_____

Current Medications

Pharmacy Contact Number: (___) ___-__

Name	Description	Dosage	Purpose

Vitamins/Food Supplements

Name	Description	Dosage	Purpose

Known Conditions, Events, and Previous Surgeries

Date	Event

NAME: _____

Personal Information

Full Name: _____ SSN: __-__-__

Address: _____ DOB: _/_/_

City/ST/Zip: _____ Phone: (__) __-__

In Case of Emergency

Contact: _____ Donor: Y/N

Home #: (__) __-__ Directives: _____

Mobile #: (__) __-__ _____

Insurance Carrier

Company: _____ ID #: _____

Employer: _____ Group #: _____

Habits

Smoker: _____ Drinks/WK: _____

Blood Type: _____ Allergies: _____

Current Medications

Pharmacy Contact Number: (__) __-__

Name	Description	Dosage	Purpose

Vitamins/Food Supplements

Name	Description	Dosage	Purpose

Known Conditions, Events, and Previous Surgeries

Date	Event

NAME: _____

Personal Information

Full Name: _____   **SSN:** __-__-__

Address: _____   **DOB:** __/__/__

City/ST/Zip: _____   **Phone:** (___) ___-___

In Case of Emergency

Contact: _____   **Donor:** Y/N

Home #: (___) ___-___   **Directives:** _____

Mobile #: (___) ___-___   _____

Insurance Carrier

Company: _____   **ID #:** _____

Employer: _____   **Group #:** _____

Habits

Smoker: _____   **Drinks/WK:** _____

Blood Type: _____   **Allergies:** _____

Current Medications

Pharmacy Contact Number: (___) ___-___

Name	Description	Dosage	Purpose

Vitamins/Food Supplements

Name	Description	Dosage	Purpose

Known Conditions, Events, and Previous Surgeries

Date	Event

NAME: _____

Personal Information

Full Name: _____   SSN: ___-__-___

Address: _____   DOB: __/__/__

City/ST/Zip: _____   Phone: (___) ___-___

In Case of Emergency

Contact: _____   Donor: Y/N

Home #: (___) ___-___   Directives: _____

Mobile #: (___) ___-___   _____

Insurance Carrier

Company: _____   ID #: _____

Employer: _____   Group #: _____

Habits

Smoker: _____   Drinks/WK: _____

Blood Type: _____   Allergies: _____

Current Medications

Pharmacy Contact Number: (___) ___-___

Name	Description	Dosage	Purpose

Vitamins/Food Supplements

Name	Description	Dosage	Purpose

Known Conditions, Events, and Previous Surgeries

Date	Event

NAME: _____

Personal Information

Full Name:	_____	**SSN:**	__-__-__
Address:	_____	**DOB:**	_/_/_
City/ST/Zip:	_____	**Phone:**	(__) __-__

In Case of Emergency

Contact:	_____	**Donor:**	Y/N
Home #:	(__) __-__	**Directives:**	_____
Mobile #:	(__) __-__		_____

Insurance Carrier

Company:	_____	**ID #:**	_____
Employer:	_____	**Group #:**	_____

Habits

Smoker:	_____	**Drinks/WK:**	_____
Blood Type:	_____	**Allergies:**	_____

Current Medications

Pharmacy Contact Number: (__) __-__

Name	Description	Dosage	Purpose

Vitamins/Food Supplements

Name	Description	Dosage	Purpose

Known Conditions, Events, and Previous Surgeries

Date	Event

NAME: _____

Personal Information

Full Name: _____ **SSN:** __-__-__

Address: _____ **DOB:** __/__/__

City/ST/Zip: _____ **Phone:** (___) ___-__

In Case of Emergency

Contact: _____ **Donor:** Y/N

Home #: (___) ___-__ **Directives:** _____

Mobile #: (___) ___-__ _____

Insurance Carrier

Company: _____ **ID #:** _____

Employer: _____ **Group #:** _____

Habits

Smoker: _____ **Drinks/WK:** _____

Blood Type: _____ **Allergies:** _____

Current Medications

Pharmacy Contact Number: (___) ___-__

Name	Description	Dosage	Purpose

Vitamins/Food Supplements

Name	Description	Dosage	Purpose

Known Conditions, Events, and Previous Surgeries

Date	Event

NAME: _____

Personal Information

Full Name: _____   SSN: __-__-__
Address: _____   DOB: __/__/__
City/ST/Zip: _____   Phone: (___) ___-__

In Case of Emergency

Contact: _____   Donor: Y/N
Home #: (___) ___-__   Directives: _____
Mobile #: (___) ___-__   _____

Insurance Carrier

Company: _____   ID #: _____
Employer: _____   Group #: _____

Habits

Smoker: _____   Drinks/WK: _____
Blood Type: _____   Allergies: _____

Current Medications

Pharmacy Contact Number: (___) ___-___

Name	Description	Dosage	Purpose

Vitamins/Food Supplements

Name	Description	Dosage	Purpose

Known Conditions, Events, and Previous Surgeries

Date	Event

NAME: _____

Personal Information

Full Name: _____   SSN: __ - __ - __

Address: _____   DOB: __/__/__

City/ST/Zip: _____   Phone: (___) ___-__

In Case of Emergency

Contact: _____   Donor: Y/N

Home #: (___) ___-__   Directives: _____

Mobile #: (___) ___-__   _____

Insurance Carrier

Company: _____   ID #: _____

Employer: _____   Group #: _____

Habits

Smoker: _____   Drinks/WK: _____

Blood Type: _____   Allergies: _____

Current Medications

Pharmacy Contact Number: (___) ___-__

Name	Description	Dosage	Purpose

Vitamins/Food Supplements

Name	Description	Dosage	Purpose

Known Conditions, Events, and Previous Surgeries

Date	Event

NAME: _____

Personal Information

Full Name: _____	**SSN:**	__ __ - __ __ - __ __
Address: _____	**DOB:**	__ / __ / __
City/ST/Zip: _____	**Phone:**	(__) ___-__

In Case of Emergency

Contact: _____	**Donor:**	Y/N
Home #: (__) ___-__	**Directives:**	_____
Mobile #: (__) ___-__		_____

Insurance Carrier

Company: _____	**ID #:**	_____
Employer: _____	**Group #:**	_____

Habits

Smoker: _____	**Drinks/WK:**	_____
Blood Type: _____	**Allergies:**	_____

Current Medications

Pharmacy Contact Number: (__) ___-__

Name	Description	Dosage	Purpose

Vitamins/Food Supplements

Name	Description	Dosage	Purpose

Known Conditions, Events, and Previous Surgeries

Date	Event

NAME: _____

Personal Information

Full Name: _____ SSN: __ __ - __ - __

Address: _____ DOB: __ / __ / __

City/ST/Zip: _____ Phone: (__) ___ - __

In Case of Emergency

Contact: _____ Donor: Y/N

Home #: (__) ___ - __ Directives: _____

Mobile #: (__) ___ - __ _____

Insurance Carrier

Company: _____ ID #: _____

Employer: _____ Group #: _____

Habits

Smoker: _____ Drinks/WK: _____

Blood Type: _____ Allergies: _____

Current Medications

Pharmacy Contact Number: (__) ___ - __

Name	Description	Dosage	Purpose

Vitamins/Food Supplements

Name	Description	Dosage	Purpose

Known Conditions, Events, and Previous Surgeries

Date	Event

NAME: _____

Personal Information

Full Name: _____   SSN: __-__-__
Address: _____   DOB: __/__/__
City/ST/Zip: _____   Phone: (___) ___-__

In Case of Emergency

Contact: _____   Donor: Y/N
Home #: (___) ___-__   Directives: _____
Mobile #: (___) ___-__   _____

Insurance Carrier

Company: _____   ID #: _____
Employer: _____   Group #: _____

Habits

Smoker: _____   Drinks/WK: _____
Blood Type: _____   Allergies: _____

Current Medications
Pharmacy Contact Number: (___) ___-__

Name	Description	Dosage	Purpose

Vitamins/Food Supplements

Name	Description	Dosage	Purpose

Known Conditions, Events, and Previous Surgeries

Date	Event

NAME: _____

Personal Information

Full Name:	_____	SSN:	__-__-__
Address:	_____	DOB:	__/__/__
City/ST/Zip:	_____	Phone:	(__) __-__

In Case of Emergency

Contact:	_____	Donor:	Y/N
Home #:	(__) __-__	Directives:	_____
Mobile #:	(__) __-__		_____

Insurance Carrier

Company:	_____	ID #:	_____
Employer:	_____	Group #:	_____

Habits

Smoker:	_____	Drinks/WK:	_____
Blood Type:	_____	Allergies:	_____

Current Medications

Pharmacy Contact Number: (__) __-__

Name	Description	Dosage	Purpose

Vitamins/Food Supplements

Name	Description	Dosage	Purpose

Known Conditions, Events, and Previous Surgeries

Date	Event

NAME: _____

Personal Information

Full Name: _____   SSN: __ - __ - __
Address: _____   DOB: __ / __ / __
City/ST/Zip: _____   Phone: (__) ___-___

In Case of Emergency

Contact: _____   Donor: Y/N
Home #:   (__) ___-___   Directives: _____
Mobile #:   (__) ___-___   _____

Insurance Carrier

Company: _____   ID #:   _____
Employer: _____   Group #:   _____

Habits

Smoker: _____   Drinks/WK: _____
Blood Type: _____   Allergies: _____

Current Medications

Pharmacy Contact Number: (__) ___-___

Name	Description	Dosage	Purpose

Vitamins/Food Supplements

Name	Description	Dosage	Purpose

Known Conditions, Events, and Previous Surgeries

Date	Event

NAME: _____

Personal Information

Full Name: _____   SSN: __ __ - __ __ - __

Address: _____   DOB: __/__/__

City/ST/Zip: _____   Phone: (___) ___-__

In Case of Emergency

Contact: _____   Donor: Y/N

Home #: (___) ___-__   Directives: _____

Mobile #: (___) ___-__   _____

Insurance Carrier

Company: _____   ID #: _____

Employer: _____   Group #: _____

Habits

Smoker: _____   Drinks/WK: _____

Blood Type: _____   Allergies: _____

Current Medications

Pharmacy Contact Number: (___) ___-__

Name	Description	Dosage	Purpose

Vitamins/Food Supplements

Name	Description	Dosage	Purpose

Known Conditions, Events, and Previous Surgeries

Date	Event

NAME: _____

Personal Information

Full Name: _____   SSN: __-__-__
Address: _____   DOB: __/__/__
City/ST/Zip: _____   Phone: (___) ___-___

In Case of Emergency

Contact: _____   Donor: Y/N
Home #: (___) ___-___   Directives: _____
Mobile #: (___) ___-___   _____

Insurance Carrier

Company: _____   ID #: _____
Employer: _____   Group #: _____

Habits

Smoker: _____   Drinks/WK: _____
Blood Type: _____   Allergies: _____

Current Medications

Pharmacy Contact Number: (___) ___-___

Name	Description	Dosage	Purpose

Vitamins/Food Supplements

Name	Description	Dosage	Purpose

Known Conditions, Events, and Previous Surgeries

Date	Event

NAME: _____

Personal Information

Full Name: _____ SSN: __-__-__

Address: _____ DOB: __/__/__

City/ST/Zip: _____ Phone: (___) ___-__

In Case of Emergency

Contact: _____ Donor: Y/N

Home #: (___) ___-__ Directives: _____

Mobile #: (___) ___-__ _____

Insurance Carrier

Company: _____ ID #: _____

Employer: _____ Group #: _____

Habits

Smoker: _____ Drinks/WK: _____

Blood Type: _____ Allergies: _____

Current Medications

Pharmacy Contact Number: (___) ___-__

Name	Description	Dosage	Purpose

Vitamins/Food Supplements

Name	Description	Dosage	Purpose

Known Conditions, Events, and Previous Surgeries

Date	Event

NAME: _____

Personal Information

Full Name:	_____	**SSN:**	__-__-__
Address:	_____	**DOB:**	__/__/__
City/ST/Zip:	_____	**Phone:**	(__) __-__

In Case of Emergency

Contact:	_____	**Donor:**	Y/N
Home #:	(__) __-__	**Directives:**	_____
Mobile #:	(__) __-__		_____

Insurance Carrier

Company:	_____	**ID #:**	_____
Employer:	_____	**Group #:**	_____

Habits

Smoker:	_____	**Drinks/WK:**	_____
Blood Type:	_____	**Allergies:**	_____

Current Medications

Pharmacy Contact Number: (__) __-__

Name	Description	Dosage	Purpose

Vitamins/Food Supplements

Name	Description	Dosage	Purpose

Known Conditions, Events, and Previous Surgeries

Date	Event

NAME: _____

Personal Information

Full Name: _____ SSN: __ - __ - __

Address: _____ DOB: __/__/__

City/ST/Zip: _____ Phone: (___) ___-__

In Case of Emergency

Contact: _____ Donor: Y/N

Home #: (___) ___-___ Directives: _____

Mobile #: (___) ___-___ _____

Insurance Carrier

Company: _____ ID #: _____

Employer: _____ Group #: _____

Habits

Smoker: _____ Drinks/WK: _____

Blood Type: _____ Allergies: _____

Current Medications

Pharmacy Contact Number: (___) ___-___

Name	Description	Dosage	Purpose

Vitamins/Food Supplements

Name	Description	Dosage	Purpose

Known Conditions, Events, and Previous Surgeries

Date	Event

NAME: _____

Personal Information

Full Name: _____   SSN: __-__-__
Address: _____   DOB: __/__/__
City/ST/Zip: _____   Phone: (___) ___-__

In Case of Emergency

Contact: _____   Donor: Y/N
Home #: (___) ___-__   Directives: _____
Mobile #: (___) ___-__   _____

Insurance Carrier

Company: _____   ID #: _____
Employer: _____   Group #: _____

Habits

Smoker: _____   Drinks/WK: _____
Blood Type: _____   Allergies: _____

Current Medications

Pharmacy Contact Number: (___) ___-___

Name	Description	Dosage	Purpose

Vitamins/Food Supplements

Name	Description	Dosage	Purpose

Known Conditions, Events, and Previous Surgeries

Date	Event

NAME: _____

Personal Information

Full Name: _____ SSN: __ - __ - __

Address: _____ DOB: __/__/__

City/ST/Zip: _____ Phone: (___) ___-___

In Case of Emergency

Contact: _____ Donor: Y/N

Home #: (___) ___-___ Directives: _____

Mobile #: (___) ___-___ _____

Insurance Carrier

Company: _____ ID #: _____

Employer: _____ Group #: _____

Habits

Smoker: _____ Drinks/WK: _____

Blood Type: _____ Allergies: _____

Current Medications

Pharmacy Contact Number: (___) ___-___

Name	Description	Dosage	Purpose

Vitamins/Food Supplements

Name	Description	Dosage	Purpose

Known Conditions, Events, and Previous Surgeries

Date	Event

NAME: _____

Personal Information

Full Name: _____   SSN: __ - __ - __

Address: _____   DOB: __/__/__

City/ST/Zip: _____   Phone: (__) __-__

In Case of Emergency

Contact: _____   Donor: Y/N

Home #: (__) __-__   Directives: _____

Mobile #: (__) __-__   _____

Insurance Carrier

Company: _____   ID #: _____

Employer: _____   Group #: _____

Habits

Smoker: _____   Drinks/WK: _____

Blood Type: _____   Allergies: _____

Current Medications

Pharmacy Contact Number: (__) __-__

Name	Description	Dosage	Purpose

Vitamins/Food Supplements

Name	Description	Dosage	Purpose

Known Conditions, Events, and Previous Surgeries

Date	Event

NAME: _____

Personal Information

Full Name: _____   SSN: __ __ - __ __ - __ __
Address: _____   DOB: __ / __ / __
City/ST/Zip: _____   Phone: (___) ___-___

In Case of Emergency

Contact: _____   Donor: Y/N
Home #: (___) ___-___   Directives: _____
Mobile #: (___) ___-___   _____

Insurance Carrier

Company: _____   ID #: _____
Employer: _____   Group #: _____

Habits

Smoker: _____   Drinks/WK: _____
Blood Type: _____ Allergies: _____

Current Medications

Pharmacy Contact Number: (___) ___-___

Name	Description	Dosage	Purpose

Vitamins/Food Supplements

Name	Description	Dosage	Purpose

Known Conditions, Events, and Previous Surgeries

Date	Event

NAME: _____

Personal Information

Full Name:	_____	SSN:	__ - __ - __
Address:	_____	DOB:	__/__/__
City/ST/Zip:	_____	Phone:	(___) ___-___

In Case of Emergency

Contact:	_____	Donor:	Y/N
Home #:	(___) ___-___	Directives:	_____
Mobile #:	(___) ___-___		_____

Insurance Carrier

Company:	_____	ID #:	_____
Employer:	_____	Group #:	_____

Habits

Smoker:	_____	Drinks/WK:	_____
Blood Type:	_____	Allergies:	_____

Current Medications

Pharmacy Contact Number: (___) ___-___

Name	Description	Dosage	Purpose

Vitamins/Food Supplements

Name	Description	Dosage	Purpose

Known Conditions, Events, and Previous Surgeries

Date	Event

NAME: _____

Personal Information

Full Name: _____   **SSN:** __-__-__
Address: _____   **DOB:** __/__/__
City/ST/Zip: _____   **Phone:** (__) __-__

In Case of Emergency

Contact: _____   **Donor:** Y/N
Home #: (__) __-__   **Directives:** _____
Mobile #: (__) __-__   _____

Insurance Carrier

Company: _____   **ID #:** _____
Employer: _____   **Group #:** _____

Habits

Smoker: _____   **Drinks/WK:** _____
Blood Type: _____   **Allergies:** _____

Current Medications

Pharmacy Contact Number: (__) __-__

Name	Description	Dosage	Purpose

Vitamins/Food Supplements

Name	Description	Dosage	Purpose

Known Conditions, Events, and Previous Surgeries

Date	Event

NAME: _____

Personal Information

Full Name:	_____	**SSN:**	__-__-__
Address:	_____	**DOB:**	__/__/__
City/ST/Zip:	_____	**Phone:**	(__) __-__

In Case of Emergency

Contact:	_____	**Donor:**	Y/N
Home #:	(__) __-__	**Directives:**	_____
Mobile #:	(__) __-__		_____

Insurance Carrier

Company:	_____	**ID #:**	_____
Employer:	_____	**Group #:**	_____

Habits

Smoker:	_____	**Drinks/WK:**	_____
Blood Type:	_____	**Allergies:**	_____

Current Medications

Pharmacy Contact Number: (__) __-__

Name	Description	Dosage	Purpose

Vitamins/Food Supplements

Name	Description	Dosage	Purpose

Known Conditions, Events, and Previous Surgeries

Date	Event

NAME: _____

Personal Information

Full Name: _____   SSN: __-__-__
Address: _____   DOB: __/__/__
City/ST/Zip: _____   Phone: (___) ___-__

In Case of Emergency

Contact: _____   Donor: Y/N
Home #: (___) ___-__   Directives: _____
Mobile #: (___) ___-__   _____

Insurance Carrier

Company: _____   ID #:   _____
Employer: _____   Group #: _____

Habits

Smoker: _____   Drinks/WK: _____
Blood Type: _____   Allergies: _____

Current Medications

Pharmacy Contact Number: (___) ___-__

Name	Description	Dosage	Purpose

Vitamins/Food Supplements

Name	Description	Dosage	Purpose

Known Conditions, Events, and Previous Surgeries

Date	Event

NAME: _____

Personal Information

Full Name: _____   SSN: __-__-__

Address: _____   DOB: __/__/__

City/ST/Zip: _____   Phone: (___) ___-___

In Case of Emergency

Contact: _____   Donor: Y/N

Home #: (___) ___-___   Directives: _____

Mobile #: (___) ___-___   _____

Insurance Carrier

Company: _____   ID #: _____

Employer: _____   Group #: _____

Habits

Smoker: _____   Drinks/WK: _____

Blood Type: _____   Allergies: _____

Current Medications

Pharmacy Contact Number: (___) ___-___

Name	Description	Dosage	Purpose

Vitamins/Food Supplements

Name	Description	Dosage	Purpose

Known Conditions, Events, and Previous Surgeries

Date	Event

NAME: _____

Personal Information

Full Name: _____ SSN: __-__-__

Address: _____ DOB: __/__/__

City/ST/Zip: _____ Phone: (___) ___-__

In Case of Emergency

Contact: _____ Donor: Y/N

Home #: (___) ___-__ Directives: _____

Mobile #: (___) ___-__ _____

Insurance Carrier

Company: _____ ID #: _____

Employer: _____ Group #: _____

Habits

Smoker: _____ Drinks/WK: _____

Blood Type: _____ Allergies: _____

Current Medications

Pharmacy Contact Number: (___) ___-__

Name	Description	Dosage	Purpose

Vitamins/Food Supplements

Name	Description	Dosage	Purpose

Known Conditions, Events, and Previous Surgeries

Date	Event

NAME: _____

Personal Information

Full Name: _____   SSN: __ - __ - __

Address: _____   DOB: __/__/__

City/ST/Zip: _____   Phone: (___) ___-___

In Case of Emergency

Contact: _____   Donor: Y/N

Home #:   (___) ___-___   Directives: _____

Mobile #:   (___) ___-___   _____

Insurance Carrier

Company: _____   ID #:   _____

Employer: _____   Group #:   _____

Habits

Smoker: _____   Drinks/WK: _____

Blood Type: _____   Allergies: _____

Current Medications

Pharmacy Contact Number: (___) ___-___

Name	Description	Dosage	Purpose

Vitamins/Food Supplements

Name	Description	Dosage	Purpose

Known Conditions, Events, and Previous Surgeries

Date	Event

NAME: _____

Personal Information

Full Name: _____   SSN: __-__-__

Address: _____   DOB: __/__/__

City/ST/Zip: _____   Phone: (___) ___-__

In Case of Emergency

Contact: _____   Donor: Y/N

Home #: (___) ___-__   Directives: _____

Mobile #: (___) ___-__   _____

Insurance Carrier

Company: _____   ID #: _____

Employer: _____   Group #: _____

Habits

Smoker: _____   Drinks/WK: _____

Blood Type: _____   Allergies: _____

Current Medications

Pharmacy Contact Number: (___) ___-__

Name	Description	Dosage	Purpose

Vitamins/Food Supplements

Name	Description	Dosage	Purpose

Known Conditions, Events, and Previous Surgeries

Date	Event

NAME: _____

Personal Information

Full Name: _____	SSN: __-__-__
Address: _____	DOB: __/__/__
City/ST/Zip: _____	Phone: (__) __-__

In Case of Emergency

Contact: _____	Donor: Y/N
Home #: (__) __-__	Directives: _____
Mobile #: (__) __-__	_____

Insurance Carrier

Company: _____	ID #: _____
Employer: _____	Group #: _____

Habits

Smoker: _____	Drinks/WK: _____
Blood Type: _____	Allergies: _____

Current Medications

Pharmacy Contact Number: (__) __-__

Name	Description	Dosage	Purpose

Vitamins/Food Supplements

Name	Description	Dosage	Purpose

Known Conditions, Events, and Previous Surgeries

Date	Event

NAME: _____

Personal Information

Full Name: _____   SSN: ___-__-__

Address: _____   DOB: __/__/__

City/ST/Zip: _____   Phone: (___) ___-__

In Case of Emergency

Contact: _____   Donor: Y/N

Home #: (___) ___-__   Directives: _____

Mobile #: (___) ___-___   _____

Insurance Carrier

Company: _____   ID #: _____

Employer: _____   Group #: _____

Habits

Smoker: _____   Drinks/WK: _____

Blood Type: _____   Allergies: _____

Current Medications

Pharmacy Contact Number: (___) ___-___

Name	Description	Dosage	Purpose

Vitamins/Food Supplements

Name	Description	Dosage	Purpose

Known Conditions, Events, and Previous Surgeries

Date	Event

NAME: _____

Personal Information

Full Name:	_____	**SSN:**	__ - __ - __
Address:	_____	**DOB:**	__/__/__
City/ST/Zip:	_____	**Phone:**	(___) ___-___

In Case of Emergency

Contact:	_____	**Donor:**	Y/N
Home #:	(___) ___-___	**Directives:**	_____
Mobile #:	(___) ___-___		_____

Insurance Carrier

Company:	_____	**ID #:**	_____
Employer:	_____	**Group #:**	_____

Habits

Smoker:	_____	**Drinks/WK:**	_____
Blood Type:	_____	**Allergies:**	_____

Current Medications

Pharmacy Contact Number: (___) ___-___

Name	Description	Dosage	Purpose

Vitamins/Food Supplements

Name	Description	Dosage	Purpose

Known Conditions, Events, and Previous Surgeries

Date	Event

NAME: _____

Personal Information

Full Name: _____   SSN: __ _ - __ - __
Address: _____   DOB: __/__/__
City/ST/Zip: _____ Phone: (___) ___-__

In Case of Emergency

Contact: _____   Donor: Y/N
Home #: (___) ___-__   Directives: _____
Mobile #: (___) ___-__   _____

Insurance Carrier

Company: _____   ID #: _____
Employer: _____   Group #: _____

Habits

Smoker: _____   Drinks/WK: _____
Blood Type: _____ Allergies: _____

Current Medications

Pharmacy Contact Number: (___) ___-__

Name	Description	Dosage	Purpose

Vitamins/Food Supplements

Name	Description	Dosage	Purpose

Known Conditions, Events, and Previous Surgeries

Date	Event

NAME: _____

Personal Information

Full Name:	_____	**SSN:**	__-__-__
Address:	_____	**DOB:**	__/__/__
City/ST/Zip:	_____	**Phone:**	(___) ___-__

In Case of Emergency

Contact:	_____	**Donor:**	Y/N
Home #:	(___) ___-__	**Directives:**	_____
Mobile #:	(___) ___-__		_____

Insurance Carrier

Company:	_____	**ID #:**	_____
Employer:	_____	**Group #:**	_____

Habits

Smoker:	_____	**Drinks/WK:**	_____
Blood Type:	_____	**Allergies:**	_____

Current Medications

Pharmacy Contact Number: (___) ___-__

Name	Description	Dosage	Purpose

Vitamins/Food Supplements

Name	Description	Dosage	Purpose

Known Conditions, Events, and Previous Surgeries

Date	Event

NAME: _____

Personal Information

Full Name:	_____	**SSN:**	__-__-__
Address:	_____	**DOB:**	__/__/__
City/ST/Zip:	_____	**Phone:**	(___) ___-__

In Case of Emergency

Contact:	_____	**Donor:**	Y/N
Home #:	(___) ___-__	**Directives:**	_____
Mobile #:	(___) ___-__		_____

Insurance Carrier

Company:	_____	**ID #:**	_____
Employer:	_____	**Group #:**	_____

Habits

Smoker:	_____	**Drinks/WK:**	_____
Blood Type:	_____	**Allergies:**	_____

Current Medications

Pharmacy Contact Number: (___) ___-__

Name	Description	Dosage	Purpose

Vitamins/Food Supplements

Name	Description	Dosage	Purpose

Known Conditions, Events, and Previous Surgeries

Date	Event

NAME: _____

Personal Information

Full Name: _____ SSN: __ - __ - __

Address: _____ DOB: __ / __ / __

City/ST/Zip: _____ Phone: (__) ___-___

In Case of Emergency

Contact: _____ Donor: Y/N

Home #: (__) ___-___ Directives: _____

Mobile #: (__) ___-___ _____

Insurance Carrier

Company: _____ ID #: _____

Employer: _____ Group #: _____

Habits

Smoker: _____ Drinks/WK: _____

Blood Type: _____ Allergies: _____

Current Medications

Pharmacy Contact Number: (__) ___-___

Name	Description	Dosage	Purpose

Vitamins/Food Supplements

Name	Description	Dosage	Purpose

Known Conditions, Events, and Previous Surgeries

Date	Event

NAME: _____

Personal Information

Full Name:	_____	**SSN:**	__ - __ - __
Address:	_____	**DOB:**	__ / __ / __
City/ST/Zip:	_____	**Phone:**	(___) ___-__

In Case of Emergency

Contact:	_____	**Donor:**	Y/N
Home #:	(___) ___-__	**Directives:**	_____
Mobile #:	(___) ___-__		_____

Insurance Carrier

Company:	_____	**ID #:**	_____
Employer:	_____	**Group #:**	_____

Habits

Smoker:	_____	**Drinks/WK:**	_____
Blood Type:	_____	**Allergies:**	_____

Current Medications

Pharmacy Contact Number: (___) ___-__

Name	Description	Dosage	Purpose

Vitamins/Food Supplements

Name	Description	Dosage	Purpose

Known Conditions, Events, and Previous Surgeries

Date	Event

NAME: _____

Personal Information

Full Name:	_____	SSN:	__-__-__
Address:	_____	DOB:	__/__/__
City/ST/Zip:	_____	Phone:	(__) __-__

In Case of Emergency

Contact:	_____	Donor:	Y/N
Home #:	(__) __-__	Directives:	_____
Mobile #:	(__) __-__		_____

Insurance Carrier

Company:	_____	ID #:	_____
Employer:	_____	Group #:	_____

Habits

Smoker:	_____	Drinks/WK:	_____
Blood Type:	_____	Allergies:	_____

Current Medications

Pharmacy Contact Number: (__) __-__

Name	Description	Dosage	Purpose

Vitamins/Food Supplements

Name	Description	Dosage	Purpose

Known Conditions, Events, and Previous Surgeries

Date	Event

NAME: _____

Personal Information

Full Name: _____ SSN: __ - __ - __

Address: _____ DOB: __/__/__

City/ST/Zip: _____ Phone: (___) ___-__

In Case of Emergency

Contact: _____ Donor: Y/N

Home #: (___) ___-__ Directives: _____

Mobile #: (___) ___-__ _____

Insurance Carrier

Company: _____ ID #: _____

Employer: _____ Group #: _____

Habits

Smoker: _____ Drinks/WK: _____

Blood Type: _____ Allergies: _____

Current Medications

Pharmacy Contact Number: (___) ___-__

Name	Description	Dosage	Purpose

Vitamins/Food Supplements

Name	Description	Dosage	Purpose

Known Conditions, Events, and Previous Surgeries

Date	Event

NAME: _____

Personal Information

Full Name: _____   SSN: __-__-__
Address: _____   DOB: __/__/__
City/ST/Zip: _____   Phone: (___) ___-___

In Case of Emergency

Contact: _____   Donor: Y/N
Home #: (___) ___-___   Directives: _____
Mobile #: (___) ___-___   _____

Insurance Carrier

Company: _____   ID #: _____
Employer: _____   Group #: _____

Habits

Smoker: _____   Drinks/WK: _____
Blood Type: _____   Allergies: _____

Current Medications

Pharmacy Contact Number: (___) ___-___

Name	Description	Dosage	Purpose

Vitamins/Food Supplements

Name	Description	Dosage	Purpose

Known Conditions, Events, and Previous Surgeries

Date	Event

NAME: _____

Personal Information

Full Name: _____   SSN: __ - __ - __

Address: _____   DOB: __/__/__

City/ST/Zip: _____   Phone: (___) ___-__

In Case of Emergency

Contact: _____   Donor: Y/N

Home #: (___) ___-__   Directives: _____

Mobile #: (___) ___-__   _____

Insurance Carrier

Company: _____   ID #: _____

Employer: _____   Group #: _____

Habits

Smoker: _____   Drinks/WK: _____

Blood Type: _____   Allergies: _____

Current Medications

Pharmacy Contact Number: (___) ___-__

Name	Description	Dosage	Purpose

Vitamins/Food Supplements

Name	Description	Dosage	Purpose

Known Conditions, Events, and Previous Surgeries

Date	Event

NAME: _____

Personal Information

Full Name: _____   SSN: ___-__-___
Address: _____   DOB: __/__/__
City/ST/Zip: _____   Phone: (___) ___-___

In Case of Emergency

Contact: _____   Donor: Y/N
Home #: (___) ___-___   Directives: _____
Mobile #: (___) ___-___   _____

Insurance Carrier

Company: _____   ID #: _____
Employer: _____   Group #: _____

Habits

Smoker: _____   Drinks/WK: _____
Blood Type: _____   Allergies: _____

Current Medications

Pharmacy Contact Number: (___) ___-___

Name	Description	Dosage	Purpose

Vitamins/Food Supplements

Name	Description	Dosage	Purpose

Known Conditions, Events, and Previous Surgeries

Date	Event

NAME: _____

Personal Information

Full Name:	_____	**SSN:**	__ - __ - __
Address:	_____	**DOB:**	__/__/__
City/ST/Zip:	_____	**Phone:**	(___) ___-___

In Case of Emergency

Contact:	_____	**Donor:**	Y/N
Home #:	(___) ___-___	**Directives:**	_____
Mobile #:	(___) ___-___		_____

Insurance Carrier

Company:	_____	**ID #:**	_____
Employer:	_____	**Group #:**	_____

Habits

Smoker:	_____	**Drinks/WK:**	_____
Blood Type:	_____	**Allergies:**	_____

Current Medications

Pharmacy Contact Number: (___) ___-___

Name	Description	Dosage	Purpose

Vitamins/Food Supplements

Name	Description	Dosage	Purpose

Known Conditions, Events, and Previous Surgeries

Date	Event

NAME: _____

Personal Information

Full Name: _____   SSN: __-__-__
Address: _____   DOB: __/__/__
City/ST/Zip: _____   Phone: (___) ___-___

In Case of Emergency

Contact: _____   Donor: Y/N
Home #: (___) ___-___   Directives: _____
Mobile #: (___) ___-___   _____

Insurance Carrier

Company: _____   ID #: _____
Employer: _____   Group #: _____

Habits

Smoker: _____   Drinks/WK: _____
Blood Type: _____   Allergies: _____

Current Medications

Pharmacy Contact Number: (___) ___-___

Name	Description	Dosage	Purpose

Vitamins/Food Supplements

Name	Description	Dosage	Purpose

Known Conditions, Events, and Previous Surgeries

Date	Event

NAME: _____

Personal Information

Full Name: _____   SSN: ___-__-___
Address: _____   DOB: __/__/__
City/ST/Zip: _____   Phone: (___) ___-___

In Case of Emergency

Contact: _____   Donor: Y/N
Home #: (___) ___-___   Directives: _____
Mobile #: (___) ___-___   _____

Insurance Carrier

Company: _____   ID #: _____
Employer: _____   Group #: _____

Habits

Smoker: _____   Drinks/WK: _____
Blood Type: _____   Allergies: _____

Current Medications

Pharmacy Contact Number: (___) ___-___

Name	Description	Dosage	Purpose

Vitamins/Food Supplements

Name	Description	Dosage	Purpose

Known Conditions, Events, and Previous Surgeries

Date	Event

NAME: _____

Personal Information

Full Name: _____   SSN: __ __ - __ - __

Address: _____   DOB: __ / __ / __

City/ST/Zip: _____   Phone: (___) ___-___

In Case of Emergency

Contact: _____   Donor: Y/N

Home #: (___) ___-___   Directives: _____

Mobile #: (___) ___-___   _____

Insurance Carrier

Company: _____   ID #: _____

Employer: _____   Group #: _____

Habits

Smoker: _____   Drinks/WK: _____

Blood Type: _____   Allergies: _____

Current Medications

Pharmacy Contact Number: (___) ___-___

Name	Description	Dosage	Purpose

Vitamins/Food Supplements

Name	Description	Dosage	Purpose

Known Conditions, Events, and Previous Surgeries

Date	Event

NAME: _____

Personal Information

Full Name: _____   SSN: __-__-__

Address: _____   DOB: __/__/__

City/ST/Zip: _____   Phone: (___) ___-__

In Case of Emergency

Contact: _____   Donor: Y/N

Home #: (___) ___-__   Directives: _____

Mobile #: (___) ___-__   _____

Insurance Carrier

Company: _____   ID #: _____

Employer: _____   Group #: _____

Habits

Smoker: _____   Drinks/WK: _____

Blood Type: _____   Allergies: _____

Current Medications

Pharmacy Contact Number: (___) ___-__

Name	Description	Dosage	Purpose

Vitamins/Food Supplements

Name	Description	Dosage	Purpose

Known Conditions, Events, and Previous Surgeries

Date	Event

NAME: _____

Personal Information

Full Name: _____   SSN: ___-__-__
Address: _____   DOB: __/__/__
City/ST/Zip: _____   Phone: (___) ___-___

In Case of Emergency

Contact: _____   Donor: Y/N
Home #: (___) ___-___   Directives: _____
Mobile #: (___) ___-___   _____

Insurance Carrier

Company: _____   ID #: _____
Employer: _____   Group #: _____

Habits

Smoker: _____   Drinks/WK: _____
Blood Type: _____   Allergies: _____

Current Medications

Pharmacy Contact Number: (___) ___-___

Name	Description	Dosage	Purpose

Vitamins/Food Supplements

Name	Description	Dosage	Purpose

Known Conditions, Events, and Previous Surgeries

Date	Event

NAME: _____

Personal Information

Full Name: _____   SSN: __ - __ - __
Address: _____   DOB: __/__/__
City/ST/Zip: _____   Phone: (___) ___-___

In Case of Emergency

Contact: _____   Donor: Y/N
Home #: (___) ___-___   Directives: _____
Mobile #: (___) ___-___   _____

Insurance Carrier

Company: _____   ID #: _____
Employer: _____   Group #: _____

Habits

Smoker: _____   Drinks/WK: _____
Blood Type: _____   Allergies: _____

Current Medications

Pharmacy Contact Number: (___) ___-___

Name	Description	Dosage	Purpose

Vitamins/Food Supplements

Name	Description	Dosage	Purpose

Known Conditions, Events, and Previous Surgeries

Date	Event

NAME: _____

Personal Information

Full Name: _____   SSN: __-__-__

Address: _____   DOB: __/__/__

City/ST/Zip: _____   Phone: (___) ___-___

In Case of Emergency

Contact: _____   Donor: Y/N

Home #: (___) ___-___   Directives: _____

Mobile #: (___) ___-___   _____

Insurance Carrier

Company: _____   ID #: _____

Employer: _____   Group #: _____

Habits

Smoker: _____   Drinks/WK: _____

Blood Type: _____   Allergies: _____

Current Medications

Pharmacy Contact Number: (___) ___-___

Name	Description	Dosage	Purpose

Vitamins/Food Supplements

Name	Description	Dosage	Purpose

Known Conditions, Events, and Previous Surgeries

Date	Event

NAME: _____

Personal Information

Full Name:	_____	**SSN:**	__ - __ - __
Address:	_____	**DOB:**	__ / __ / __
City/ST/Zip:	_____	**Phone:**	(___) ___ - ___

In Case of Emergency

Contact:	_____	**Donor:**	Y/N
Home #:	(___) ___ - ___	**Directives:**	_____
Mobile #:	(___) ___ - ___		_____

Insurance Carrier

Company:	_____	**ID #:**	_____
Employer:	_____	**Group #:**	_____

Habits

Smoker:	_____	**Drinks/WK:**	_____
Blood Type:	_____	**Allergies:**	_____

Current Medications

Pharmacy Contact Number: (___) ___ - ___

Name	Description	Dosage	Purpose

Vitamins/Food Supplements

Name	Description	Dosage	Purpose

Known Conditions, Events, and Previous Surgeries

Date	Event

NAME: _____

Personal Information

Full Name: _____   SSN: __-__-__

Address: _____   DOB: __/__/__

City/ST/Zip: _____   Phone: (___) ___-___

In Case of Emergency

Contact: _____   Donor: Y/N

Home #: (___) ___-___   Directives: _____

Mobile #: (___) ___-___   _____

Insurance Carrier

Company: _____   ID #: _____

Employer: _____   Group #: _____

Habits

Smoker: _____   Drinks/WK: _____

Blood Type: _____   Allergies: _____

Current Medications

Pharmacy Contact Number: (___) ___-___

Name	Description	Dosage	Purpose

Vitamins/Food Supplements

Name	Description	Dosage	Purpose

Known Conditions, Events, and Previous Surgeries

Date	Event

NAME: _____

Personal Information

Full Name:	_____	**SSN:**	__ - __ - __
Address:	_____	**DOB:**	__ / __ / __
City/ST/Zip:	_____	**Phone:**	(___) ___ - __

In Case of Emergency

Contact:	_____	**Donor:**	Y/N
Home #:	(___) ___ - __	**Directives:**	_____
Mobile #:	(___) ___ - __		_____

Insurance Carrier

Company:	_____	**ID #:**	_____
Employer:	_____	**Group #:**	_____

Habits

Smoker:	_____	**Drinks/WK:**	_____
Blood Type:	_____	**Allergies:**	_____

Current Medications

Pharmacy Contact Number: (___) ___ - __

Name	Description	Dosage	Purpose

Vitamins/Food Supplements

Name	Description	Dosage	Purpose

Known Conditions, Events, and Previous Surgeries

Date	Event

NAME: _____

Personal Information

Full Name: _____   SSN: __-__-__
Address: _____   DOB: __/__/__
City/ST/Zip: _____   Phone: (___) ___-__

In Case of Emergency

Contact: _____   Donor: Y/N
Home #: (___) ___-__   Directives: _____
Mobile #: (___) ___-__   _____

Insurance Carrier

Company: _____   ID #: _____
Employer: _____   Group #: _____

Habits

Smoker: _____   Drinks/WK: _____
Blood Type: _____   Allergies: _____

Current Medications
Pharmacy Contact Number: (___) ___-__

Name	Description	Dosage	Purpose

Vitamins/Food Supplements

Name	Description	Dosage	Purpose

Known Conditions, Events, and Previous Surgeries

Date	Event

NAME: _____

Personal Information

Full Name: _____   SSN: __ __ - __ __ - __

Address: _____   DOB: __ / __ / __

City/ST/Zip: _____   Phone: (__) __ - __

In Case of Emergency

Contact: _____   Donor: Y/N

Home #: (__) __ - __   Directives: _____

Mobile #: (__) __ - __   _____

Insurance Carrier

Company: _____   ID #: _____

Employer: _____   Group #: _____

Habits

Smoker: _____   Drinks/WK: _____

Blood Type: _____   Allergies: _____

Current Medications

Pharmacy Contact Number: (__) __ - __

Name	Description	Dosage	Purpose

Vitamins/Food Supplements

Name	Description	Dosage	Purpose

Known Conditions, Events, and Previous Surgeries

Date	Event

NAME: _____

Personal Information

Full Name: _____   SSN: __ - __ - __
Address: _____   DOB: __/__/__
City/ST/Zip: _____   Phone: (___) ___-___

In Case of Emergency

Contact: _____   Donor: Y/N
Home #: (___) ___-___   Directives: _____
Mobile #: (___) ___-___   _____

Insurance Carrier

Company: _____   ID #: _____
Employer: _____   Group #: _____

Habits

Smoker: _____   Drinks/WK: _____
Blood Type: _____   Allergies: _____

Current Medications

Pharmacy Contact Number: (___) ___-___

Name	Description	Dosage	Purpose

Vitamins/Food Supplements

Name	Description	Dosage	Purpose

Known Conditions, Events, and Previous Surgeries

Date	Event

NAME: _____

Personal Information

Full Name: _____   SSN: __-__-__
Address: _____   DOB: __/__/__
City/ST/Zip: _____   Phone: (___) ___-__

In Case of Emergency

Contact: _____   Donor: Y/N
Home #: (___) ___-__   Directives: _____
Mobile #: (___) ___-__   _____

Insurance Carrier

Company: _____   ID #: _____
Employer: _____   Group #: _____

Habits

Smoker: _____   Drinks/WK: _____
Blood Type: _____   Allergies: _____

Current Medications

Pharmacy Contact Number: (___) ___-__

Name	Description	Dosage	Purpose

Vitamins/Food Supplements

Name	Description	Dosage	Purpose

Known Conditions, Events, and Previous Surgeries

Date	Event

NAME: _____

Personal Information

Full Name: _____   SSN: ___-__-__
Address: _____   DOB: __/__/__
City/ST/Zip: _____   Phone: (___) ___-___

In Case of Emergency

Contact: _____   Donor: Y/N
Home #: (___) ___-___   Directives: _____
Mobile #: (___) ___-___   _____

Insurance Carrier

Company: _____   ID #: _____
Employer: _____   Group #: _____

Habits

Smoker: _____   Drinks/WK: _____
Blood Type: _____   Allergies: _____

Current Medications

Pharmacy Contact Number: (___) ___-___

Name	Description	Dosage	Purpose

Vitamins/Food Supplements

Name	Description	Dosage	Purpose

Known Conditions, Events, and Previous Surgeries

Date	Event

NAME: _____

Personal Information

Full Name:	_____	**SSN:**	__-__-__
Address:	_____	**DOB:**	__/__/__
City/ST/Zip:	_____	**Phone:**	(___) ___-___

In Case of Emergency

Contact:	_____	**Donor:**	Y/N
Home #:	(___) ___-___	**Directives:**	_____
Mobile #:	(___) ___-___		_____

Insurance Carrier

Company:	_____	**ID #:**	_____
Employer:	_____	**Group #:**	_____

Habits

Smoker:	_____	**Drinks/WK:**	_____
Blood Type:	_____	**Allergies:**	_____

Current Medications

Pharmacy Contact Number: (___) ___-___

Name	Description	Dosage	Purpose

Vitamins/Food Supplements

Name	Description	Dosage	Purpose

Known Conditions, Events, and Previous Surgeries

Date	Event

NAME: _____

Personal Information

Full Name: _____	**SSN:** __ _ - __ - __
Address: _____	**DOB:** __/__/__
City/ST/Zip: _____	**Phone:** (___) ___-__

In Case of Emergency

Contact: _____	**Donor:** Y/N
Home #: (___) ___-__	**Directives:** _____
Mobile #: (___) ___-__	_____

Insurance Carrier

Company: _____	**ID #:** _____
Employer: _____	**Group #:** _____

Habits

Smoker: _____	**Drinks/WK:** _____
Blood Type: _____	**Allergies:** _____

Current Medications

Pharmacy Contact Number: (___) ___-__

Name	Description	Dosage	Purpose

Vitamins/Food Supplements

Name	Description	Dosage	Purpose

Known Conditions, Events, and Previous Surgeries

Date	Event

NAME: _____

Personal Information

Full Name: _____   SSN: __ _ - __ __ - __ __
Address: _____   DOB: __ / __ / __
City/ST/Zip: _____   Phone: (___) ___-__

In Case of Emergency

Contact: _____   Donor: Y/N
Home #: (___) ___-__   Directives: _____
Mobile #: (___) ___-__   _____

Insurance Carrier

Company: _____   ID #: _____
Employer: _____   Group #: _____

Habits

Smoker: _____   Drinks/WK: _____
Blood Type: _____   Allergies: _____

Current Medications

Pharmacy Contact Number: (___) ___-___

Name	Description	Dosage	Purpose

Vitamins/Food Supplements

Name	Description	Dosage	Purpose

Known Conditions, Events, and Previous Surgeries

Date	Event

NAME: _____

Personal Information

Full Name: _____ SSN: __ - __ - __

Address: _____ DOB: __/__/__

City/ST/Zip: _____ Phone: (___) ___-___

In Case of Emergency

Contact: _____ Donor: Y/N

Home #: (___) ___-___ Directives: _____

Mobile #: (___) ___-___ _____

Insurance Carrier

Company: _____ ID #: _____

Employer: _____ Group #: _____

Habits

Smoker: _____ Drinks/WK: _____

Blood Type: _____ Allergies: _____

Current Medications

Pharmacy Contact Number: (___) ___-___

Name	Description	Dosage	Purpose

Vitamins/Food Supplements

Name	Description	Dosage	Purpose

Known Conditions, Events, and Previous Surgeries

Date	Event

NAME: _____

Personal Information

Full Name:	_____	SSN:	__ - __ - __
Address:	_____	DOB:	__/__/__
City/ST/Zip:	_____	Phone:	(__) __ - __

In Case of Emergency

Contact:	_____	Donor:	Y/N
Home #:	(__) __ - __	Directives:	_____
Mobile #:	(__) __ - __		_____

Insurance Carrier

Company:	_____	ID #:	_____
Employer:	_____	Group #:	_____

Habits

Smoker:	_____	Drinks/WK:	_____
Blood Type:	_____	Allergies:	_____

Current Medications

Pharmacy Contact Number: (__) __ - __

Name	Description	Dosage	Purpose

Vitamins/Food Supplements

Name	Description	Dosage	Purpose

Known Conditions, Events, and Previous Surgeries

Date	Event

NAME: _____

Personal Information

Full Name: _____   SSN: __ - __ - __
Address: _____   DOB: __ / __ / __
City/ST/Zip: _____   Phone: (___) ___-___

In Case of Emergency

Contact: _____   Donor: Y/N
Home #: (___) ___-___   Directives: _____
Mobile #: (___) ___-___   _____

Insurance Carrier

Company: _____   ID #: _____
Employer: _____   Group #: _____

Habits

Smoker: _____   Drinks/WK: _____
Blood Type: _____   Allergies: _____

Current Medications

Pharmacy Contact Number: (___) ___-___

Name	Description	Dosage	Purpose

Vitamins/Food Supplements

Name	Description	Dosage	Purpose

Known Conditions, Events, and Previous Surgeries

Date	Event

NAME: _____

Personal Information

Full Name: _____   SSN: __-__-__
Address: _____   DOB: __/__/__
City/ST/Zip: _____   Phone: (___) ___-__

In Case of Emergency

Contact: _____   Donor: Y/N
Home #: (___) ___-__   Directives: _____
Mobile #: (___) ___-__   _____

Insurance Carrier

Company: _____   ID #: _____
Employer: _____   Group #: _____

Habits

Smoker: _____   Drinks/WK: _____
Blood Type: _____   Allergies: _____

Current Medications

Pharmacy Contact Number: (___) ___-___

Name	Description	Dosage	Purpose

Vitamins/Food Supplements

Name	Description	Dosage	Purpose

Known Conditions, Events, and Previous Surgeries

Date	Event

NAME: _____

Personal Information

Full Name:	_____	**SSN:**	__-__-__
Address:	_____	**DOB:**	_/_/_
City/ST/Zip:	_____	**Phone:**	(__) __-__

In Case of Emergency

Contact:	_____	**Donor:**	Y/N
Home #:	(__) __-__	**Directives:**	_____
Mobile #:	(__) __-__		_____

Insurance Carrier

Company:	_____	**ID #:**	_____
Employer:	_____	**Group #:**	_____

Habits

Smoker:	_____	**Drinks/WK:**	_____
Blood Type:	_____	**Allergies:**	_____

Current Medications

Pharmacy Contact Number: (__) __-__

Name	Description	Dosage	Purpose

Vitamins/Food Supplements

Name	Description	Dosage	Purpose

Known Conditions, Events, and Previous Surgeries

Date	Event

NAME: _____

Personal Information

Full Name: _____   SSN: __-__-__
Address: _____   DOB: __/__/__
City/ST/Zip: _____   Phone: (___) ___-__

In Case of Emergency

Contact: _____   Donor: Y/N
Home #: (___) ___-___   Directives: _____
Mobile #: (___) ___-___   _____

Insurance Carrier

Company: _____   ID #: _____
Employer: _____   Group #: _____

Habits

Smoker: _____   Drinks/WK: _____
Blood Type: _____   Allergies: _____

Current Medications

Pharmacy Contact Number: (___) ___-___

Name	Description	Dosage	Purpose

Vitamins/Food Supplements

Name	Description	Dosage	Purpose

Known Conditions, Events, and Previous Surgeries

Date	Event

NAME: _____

Personal Information

Full Name: _____ SSN: __-__-__

Address: _____ DOB: __/__/__

City/ST/Zip: _____ Phone: (___) ___-___

In Case of Emergency

Contact: _____ Donor: Y/N

Home #: (___) ___-___ Directives: _____

Mobile #: (___) ___-___ _____

Insurance Carrier

Company: _____ ID #: _____

Employer: _____ Group #: _____

Habits

Smoker: _____ Drinks/WK: _____

Blood Type: _____ Allergies: _____

Current Medications

Pharmacy Contact Number: (___) ___-___

Name	Description	Dosage	Purpose

Vitamins/Food Supplements

Name	Description	Dosage	Purpose

Known Conditions, Events, and Previous Surgeries

Date	Event

NAME: _____

Personal Information

Full Name: _____   SSN: __-__-__

Address: _____   DOB: __/__/__

City/ST/Zip: _____   Phone: (__) __-__

In Case of Emergency

Contact: _____   Donor: Y/N

Home #: (__) __-__   Directives: _____

Mobile #: (__) __-__   _____

Insurance Carrier

Company: _____   ID #: _____

Employer: _____   Group #: _____

Habits

Smoker: _____   Drinks/WK: _____

Blood Type: _____   Allergies: _____

Current Medications

Pharmacy Contact Number: (__) __-__

Name	Description	Dosage	Purpose

Vitamins/Food Supplements

Name	Description	Dosage	Purpose

Known Conditions, Events, and Previous Surgeries

Date	Event

NAME: _____

Personal Information

Full Name: _____   SSN: ___-___-___

Address: _____   DOB: ___/___/___

City/ST/Zip: _____   Phone: (___) ___-___

In Case of Emergency

Contact: _____   Donor: Y/N

Home #: (___) ___-___   Directives: _____

Mobile #: (___) ___-___   _____

Insurance Carrier

Company: _____   ID #: _____

Employer: _____   Group #: _____

Habits

Smoker: _____   Drinks/WK: _____

Blood Type: _____   Allergies: _____

Current Medications

Pharmacy Contact Number: (___) ___-___

Name	Description	Dosage	Purpose

Vitamins/Food Supplements

Name	Description	Dosage	Purpose

Known Conditions, Events, and Previous Surgeries

Date	Event

NAME: _____

Personal Information

Full Name: _____   **SSN:** __ - __ - __

Address: _____   **DOB:** __/__/__

City/ST/Zip: _____   **Phone:** (__) __ - __

In Case of Emergency

Contact: _____   **Donor:**   Y/N

Home #: (__) __ - __   **Directives:** _____

Mobile #: (__) __ - __   _____

Insurance Carrier

Company: _____   **ID #:** _____

Employer: _____   **Group #:** _____

Habits

Smoker: _____   **Drinks/WK:** _____

Blood Type: _____   **Allergies:** _____

Current Medications

Pharmacy Contact Number: (__) __ - __

Name	Description	Dosage	Purpose

Vitamins/Food Supplements

Name	Description	Dosage	Purpose

Known Conditions, Events, and Previous Surgeries

Date	Event

NAME: _____

Personal Information

Full Name: _____   SSN: ___-___-___
Address: _____   DOB: __/__/__
City/ST/Zip: _____   Phone: (___) ___-___

In Case of Emergency

Contact: _____   Donor: Y/N
Home #: (___) ___-___   Directives: _____
Mobile #: (___) ___-___   _____

Insurance Carrier

Company: _____   ID #: _____
Employer: _____   Group #: _____

Habits

Smoker: _____   Drinks/WK: _____
Blood Type: _____   Allergies: _____

Current Medications

Pharmacy Contact Number: (___) ___-___

Name	Description	Dosage	Purpose

Vitamins/Food Supplements

Name	Description	Dosage	Purpose

Known Conditions, Events, and Previous Surgeries

Date	Event

NAME: _____

Personal Information

Full Name: _____ SSN: __-__-__

Address: _____ DOB: __/__/__

City/ST/Zip: _____ Phone: (___) ___-___

In Case of Emergency

Contact: _____ Donor: Y/N

Home #: (___) ___-___ Directives: _____

Mobile #: (___) ___-___ _____

Insurance Carrier

Company: _____ ID #: _____

Employer: _____ Group #: _____

Habits

Smoker: _____ Drinks/WK: _____

Blood Type: _____ Allergies: _____

Current Medications

Pharmacy Contact Number: (___) ___-___

Name	Description	Dosage	Purpose

Vitamins/Food Supplements

Name	Description	Dosage	Purpose

Known Conditions, Events, and Previous Surgeries

Date	Event

NAME: _____

Personal Information

Full Name: _____	**SSN:** __-__-__
Address: _____	**DOB:** __/__/__
City/ST/Zip: _____	**Phone:** (___) ___-__

In Case of Emergency

Contact: _____	**Donor:** Y/N
Home #: (___) ___-__	**Directives:** _____
Mobile #: (___) ___-__	_____

Insurance Carrier

Company: _____	**ID #:** _____
Employer: _____	**Group #:** _____

Habits

Smoker: _____	**Drinks/WK:** _____
Blood Type: _____	**Allergies:** _____

Current Medications

Pharmacy Contact Number: (___) ___-__

Name	Description	Dosage	Purpose

Vitamins/Food Supplements

Name	Description	Dosage	Purpose

Known Conditions, Events, and Previous Surgeries

Date	Event

NAME: _____

Personal Information

Full Name: _____	**SSN:** __ - __ - __
Address: _____	**DOB:** __ / __ / __
City/ST/Zip: _____	**Phone:** (__) __ - __

In Case of Emergency

Contact: _____	**Donor:** Y/N
Home #: (__) __ - __	**Directives:** _____
Mobile #: (__) __ - __	_____

Insurance Carrier

Company: _____	**ID #:** _____
Employer: _____	**Group #:** _____

Habits

Smoker: _____	**Drinks/WK:** _____
Blood Type: _____	**Allergies:** _____

Current Medications

Pharmacy Contact Number: (__) __ - __

Name	Description	Dosage	Purpose

Vitamins/Food Supplements

Name	Description	Dosage	Purpose

Known Conditions, Events, and Previous Surgeries

Date	Event

NAME: _____

Personal Information

Full Name: _____	**SSN:** __ __ - __ __ - __ __
Address: _____	**DOB:** __ / __ / __
City/ST/Zip: _____	**Phone:** (__) __ - __

In Case of Emergency

Contact: _____	**Donor:** Y/N
Home #: (__) __ - __	**Directives:** _____
Mobile #: (__) __ - __	_____

Insurance Carrier

Company: _____	**ID #:** _____
Employer: _____	**Group #:** _____

Habits

Smoker: _____	**Drinks/WK:** _____
Blood Type: _____	**Allergies:** _____

Current Medications

Pharmacy Contact Number: (__) __ - __

Name	Description	Dosage	Purpose

Vitamins/Food Supplements

Name	Description	Dosage	Purpose

Known Conditions, Events, and Previous Surgeries

Date	Event

NAME: _____

Personal Information

Full Name: _____   SSN: __ _ - __ - __
Address: _____   DOB: __/__/__
City/ST/Zip: _____   Phone: (___) ___-___

In Case of Emergency

Contact: _____   Donor: Y/N
Home #: (___) ___-___   Directives: _____
Mobile #: (___) ___-___   _____

Insurance Carrier

Company: _____   ID #: _____
Employer: _____   Group #: _____

Habits

Smoker: _____   Drinks/WK: _____
Blood Type: _____   Allergies: _____

Current Medications
Pharmacy Contact Number: (___) ___-___

Name	Description	Dosage	Purpose

Vitamins/Food Supplements

Name	Description	Dosage	Purpose

Known Conditions, Events, and Previous Surgeries

Date	Event

NAME: _____

Personal Information

Full Name: _____   SSN: __-__-__
Address: _____   DOB: __/__/__
City/ST/Zip: _____   Phone: (___) ___-___

In Case of Emergency

Contact: _____   Donor: Y/N
Home #: (___) ___-___   Directives: _____
Mobile #: (___) ___-___   _____

Insurance Carrier

Company: _____   ID #: _____
Employer: _____   Group #: _____

Habits

Smoker: _____   Drinks/WK: _____
Blood Type: _____   Allergies: _____

Current Medications

Pharmacy Contact Number: (___) ___-___

Name	Description	Dosage	Purpose

Vitamins/Food Supplements

Name	Description	Dosage	Purpose

Known Conditions, Events, and Previous Surgeries

Date	Event

NAME: _____

Personal Information

Full Name: _____   SSN: __-__-__

Address: _____   DOB: __/__/__

City/ST/Zip: _____   Phone: (___) ___-___

In Case of Emergency

Contact: _____   Donor: Y/N

Home #: (___) ___-___   Directives: _____

Mobile #: (___) ___-___   _____

Insurance Carrier

Company: _____   ID #: _____

Employer: _____   Group #: _____

Habits

Smoker: _____   Drinks/WK: _____

Blood Type: _____   Allergies: _____

Current Medications

Pharmacy Contact Number: (___) ___-___

Name	Description	Dosage	Purpose

Vitamins/Food Supplements

Name	Description	Dosage	Purpose

Known Conditions, Events, and Previous Surgeries

Date	Event

NAME: _____

Personal Information

Full Name: _____ SSN: ___-__-__

Address: _____ DOB: __/__/__

City/ST/Zip: _____ Phone: (___) ___-__

In Case of Emergency

Contact: _____ Donor: Y/N

Home #: (___) ___-__ Directives: _____

Mobile #: (___) ___-__ _____

Insurance Carrier

Company: _____ ID #: _____

Employer: _____ Group #: _____

Habits

Smoker: _____ Drinks/WK: _____

Blood Type: _____ Allergies: _____

Current Medications

Pharmacy Contact Number: (___) ___-__

Name	Description	Dosage	Purpose

Vitamins/Food Supplements

Name	Description	Dosage	Purpose

Known Conditions, Events, and Previous Surgeries

Date	Event

NAME: _____

Personal Information

Full Name:	_____	**SSN:**	__-__-__
Address:	_____	**DOB:**	_/_/_
City/ST/Zip:	_____	**Phone:**	(__) __-__

In Case of Emergency

Contact:	_____	**Donor:**	Y/N
Home #:	(__) __-__	**Directives:**	_____
Mobile #:	(__) __-__		_____

Insurance Carrier

Company:	_____	**ID #:**	_____
Employer:	_____	**Group #:**	_____

Habits

Smoker:	_____	**Drinks/WK:**	_____
Blood Type:	_____	**Allergies:**	_____

Current Medications

Pharmacy Contact Number: (__) __-__

Name	Description	Dosage	Purpose

Vitamins/Food Supplements

Name	Description	Dosage	Purpose

Known Conditions, Events, and Previous Surgeries

Date	Event

NAME: _____

Personal Information

Full Name: _____   SSN: __-__-__

Address: _____   DOB: __/__/__

City/ST/Zip: _____   Phone: (___) ___-___

In Case of Emergency

Contact: _____   Donor: Y/N

Home #: (___) ___-___   Directives: _____

Mobile #: (___) ___-___   _____

Insurance Carrier

Company: _____   ID #: _____

Employer: _____   Group #: _____

Habits

Smoker: _____   Drinks/WK: _____

Blood Type: _____   Allergies: _____

Current Medications

Pharmacy Contact Number: (___) ___-___

Name	Description	Dosage	Purpose

Vitamins/Food Supplements

Name	Description	Dosage	Purpose

Known Conditions, Events, and Previous Surgeries

Date	Event

NAME: _____

Personal Information

Full Name: _____   SSN: __-__-__

Address: _____   DOB: __/__/__

City/ST/Zip: _____   Phone: (___) ___-___

In Case of Emergency

Contact: _____   Donor: Y/N

Home #: (___) ___-___   Directives: _____

Mobile #: (___) ___-___   _____

Insurance Carrier

Company: _____   ID #: _____

Employer: _____   Group #: _____

Habits

Smoker: _____   Drinks/WK: _____

Blood Type: _____   Allergies: _____

Current Medications

Pharmacy Contact Number: (___) ___-___

Name	Description	Dosage	Purpose

Vitamins/Food Supplements

Name	Description	Dosage	Purpose

Known Conditions, Events, and Previous Surgeries

Date	Event

NAME: _____

Personal Information

Full Name: _____ **SSN:** __-__-__

Address: _____ **DOB:** __/__/__

City/ST/Zip: _____ **Phone:** (__) __-__

In Case of Emergency

Contact: _____ **Donor:** Y/N

Home #: (__) __-__ **Directives:** _____

Mobile #: (__) __-__ _____

Insurance Carrier

Company: _____ **ID #:** _____

Employer: _____ **Group #:** _____

Habits

Smoker: _____ **Drinks/WK:** _____

Blood Type: _____ **Allergies:** _____

Current Medications

Pharmacy Contact Number: (__) __-__

Name	Description	Dosage	Purpose

Vitamins/Food Supplements

Name	Description	Dosage	Purpose

Known Conditions, Events, and Previous Surgeries

Date	Event

NAME: _____

Personal Information

Full Name:	_____	**SSN:**	__-__-__
Address:	_____	**DOB:**	__/__/__
City/ST/Zip:	_____	**Phone:**	(___) ___-__

In Case of Emergency

Contact:	_____	**Donor:**	Y/N
Home #:	(___) ___-__	**Directives:**	_____
Mobile #:	(___) ___-__		_____

Insurance Carrier

Company:	_____	**ID #:**	_____
Employer:	_____	**Group #:**	_____

Habits

Smoker:	_____	**Drinks/WK:**	_____
Blood Type:	_____	**Allergies:**	_____

Current Medications

Pharmacy Contact Number: (___) ___-__

Name	Description	Dosage	Purpose

Vitamins/Food Supplements

Name	Description	Dosage	Purpose

Known Conditions, Events, and Previous Surgeries

Date	Event

NAME: _____

Personal Information

Full Name: _____   SSN: __ - __ - __
Address: _____   DOB: __/__/__
City/ST/Zip: _____   Phone: (__) __ - __

In Case of Emergency

Contact: _____   Donor: Y/N
Home #: (__) __ - __   Directives: _____
Mobile #: (__) __ - __   _____

Insurance Carrier

Company: _____   ID #: _____
Employer: _____   Group #: _____

Habits

Smoker: _____   Drinks/WK: _____
Blood Type: _____   Allergies: _____

Current Medications
Pharmacy Contact Number: (__) __ - __

Name	Description	Dosage	Purpose

Vitamins/Food Supplements

Name	Description	Dosage	Purpose

Known Conditions, Events, and Previous Surgeries

Date	Event

NAME: _____

Personal Information

Full Name: _____	**SSN:** __ - __ - __
Address: _____	**DOB:** __/__/__
City/ST/Zip: _____	**Phone:** (__) __-__

In Case of Emergency

Contact: _____	**Donor:** Y/N
Home #: (__) __-__	**Directives:** _____
Mobile #: (__) __-__	_____

Insurance Carrier

Company: _____	**ID #:** _____
Employer: _____	**Group #:** _____

Habits

Smoker: _____	**Drinks/WK:** _____
Blood Type: _____	**Allergies:** _____

Current Medications

Pharmacy Contact Number: (__) __-__

Name	Description	Dosage	Purpose

Vitamins/Food Supplements

Name	Description	Dosage	Purpose

Known Conditions, Events, and Previous Surgeries

Date	Event

NAME: _____

Personal Information

Full Name: _____   SSN: __-__-__
Address: _____   DOB: __/__/__
City/ST/Zip: _____ Phone: (__) __-__

In Case of Emergency

Contact: _____   Donor: Y/N
Home #: (__) __-__   Directives: _____
Mobile #: (__) __-__   _____

Insurance Carrier

Company: _____   ID #: _____
Employer: _____   Group #: _____

Habits

Smoker: _____   Drinks/WK: _____
Blood Type: _____   Allergies: _____

Current Medications

Pharmacy Contact Number: (__) __-__

Name	Description	Dosage	Purpose

Vitamins/Food Supplements

Name	Description	Dosage	Purpose

Known Conditions, Events, and Previous Surgeries

Date	Event

NAME: _____

Personal Information

Full Name:	_____	**SSN:**	__ - __ - __
Address:	_____	**DOB:**	__/__/__
City/ST/Zip:	_____	**Phone:**	(__) __ - __

In Case of Emergency

Contact:	_____	**Donor:**	Y/N
Home #:	(__) __ - __	**Directives:**	_____
Mobile #:	(__) __ - __		_____

Insurance Carrier

Company:	_____	**ID #:**	_____
Employer:	_____	**Group #:**	_____

Habits

Smoker:	_____	**Drinks/WK:**	_____
Blood Type:	_____	**Allergies:**	_____

Current Medications

Pharmacy Contact Number: (__) __ - __

Name	Description	Dosage	Purpose

Vitamins/Food Supplements

Name	Description	Dosage	Purpose

Known Conditions, Events, and Previous Surgeries

Date	Event